EVERYDAY SAFETY

"Safety Strategies for Everyday Situations"

TERRY J. STONE

Table of content

Introduction to emergency preparedness

Emergency preparation is a comprehensive and proactive strategy that prepares people, families, and communities to efficiently deal with unforeseen crises and disasters. The major purpose is to mitigate the consequences of crises, increase resilience, and speed up recovery activities. This preventive approach includes a variety of activities, talents, and resources that contribute to a coordinated and successful reaction in times of disaster.

Emergency preparation is primarily about understanding and recognising possible risks and dangers. These include natural catastrophes such as earthquakes, floods, and storms, as well as human-caused occurrences such as industrial accidents or health crises like pandemics. By conducting detailed risk assessments, individuals and communities may tailor their preparation efforts to successfully handle the specific difficulties they may face.

Comprehensive disaster planning and the establishment of well-stocked emergency kits are critical steps towards readiness. These kits often include necessary goods such as non-perishable food, water, prescriptions, first aid supplies, and important papers. Continuously reviewing and maintaining these kits ensures that persons have the necessary materials to survive the critical early stages of any emergency crisis.

Emergency preparation relies heavily on clear and effective communication. Establishing good communication channels across families, businesses, and communities is critical for successfully disseminating information and coordinating response actions during an emergency. This requires creating thorough communication strategies that detail the techniques and processes for exchanging and receiving information in crucial circumstances.

Emergency preparation should not be seen as an individual endeavour, but as a shared responsibility. By actively engaging the community, collaborating with local authorities, and participating in broader efforts, we can improve our response network and efficiently solve unanticipated issues. This collaborative approach improves our capacity to overcome adversity, making the environment safer and more secure for all parties involved.

Basic first aid skills

Having a solid understanding of basic first aid skills is essential when it comes to promptly aiding individuals who experience sudden illness or injury. These skills hold great importance in facilitating recovery and minimizing further harm prior to the arrival of medical professionals. Let's explore a few fundamental first aid skills that everyone should be familiar with.

Assessment of the situation:

- To guarantee the safety of individuals involved, including yourself, the affected person, and any onlookers.
- Before you approach the injured individual, it is crucial to evaluate the surroundings for any possible dangers or risks that may be present.

Calling for help

- If the circumstances necessitate the expertise of medical professionals, it is imperative to promptly contact emergency services.

CPR (cardiopulmonary resuscitation):

- Performing CPR is a crucial skill that entails administering chest compressions and rescue breaths to sustain blood flow and oxygenation during instances of cardiac arrest. Gain vital knowledge on CPR, including techniques for maintaining circulation and oxygen in emergency situations.

Choking responses:

- Familiarize yourself with the Heimlich maneuver, which is used to clear a blocked airway in conscious individuals.

- Learn the proper technique for administering chest thrusts to infants when they are choking.

Control of bleeding:

- Apply firm pressure to injuries by utilizing a sanitary fabric or dressing.
- If feasible, raise the wounded limb to minimize the circulation of blood.
- When faced with severe bleeding, it is advisable to consider using a tourniquet only as a final measure.

Treating burns:

- It is recommended to use cold running water to cool burns for a minimum of 10 minutes.
- When dealing with burns, it is important to carefully apply a sterile dressing that does not stick to the skin. This will help protect the affected

Effective Techniques for Handling Fractures and Sprains

- To prevent further harm, it is crucial to immobilize the injured limb by applying a splint or bandage.
- Elevate the injured limb to reduce swelling.

Recognizing and responding to shock:

- Lay the individual down and hoist their legs marginally, unless there are suspected head, neck , back or leg wounds.
- Keep the individual warm and consoled..

Managing with minor wounds:

- Clean and dress little wounds to anticipate disease.

- Apply ice packs to decrease swelling in minor wounds

Seizure reaction:

- Ensure the individual from harm by moving objects absent.
- Don't control the individual, but direct them tenderly to the ground and put their side after the seizure.

Recognizing signs of heart attack or strokes:

- Be commonplace with the signs and side effects of a heart assault or stroke.
- Energize the individual to sit down and look for therapeutic offer assistance instantly.

Utilize of AED (mechanized outside defibrillator):

- On the off chance that prepared, utilize an AED in case of sudden cardiac capture.

Keep in mind that these fundamental to begin with help aptitudes are not a substitute for proficient therapeutic care. Continuously look for proficient offer assistance for genuine wounds or restorative crisis. moreover , consider taking a certified to begin with help and CPR course to improve your abilities and certainty in giving help in crisis circumstances.

Recognizing and responding to medical emergencies

Recognizing and responding to medical emergencies requires a combination of awareness, prompt action, and appropriate interventions. Here are general guidelines for recognizing and responding to common medical emergencies:

1. Heart Attack:

Recognition:

- Chest discomfort, pain, or pressure.
- Shortness of breath.
- Sweating, nausea, or lightheadedness.

Response:

- Call emergency services immediately.
- Have the person sit down and rest.

- If they have prescribed medication (such as nitroglycerin), assist in taking it.

2. Stroke:

- Recognition:
- Sudden numbness or weakness, especially on one side of the body.
- Confusion, trouble speaking, or difficulty understanding speech.
- Severe headache.

Response:

- Call emergency services immediately.
- Keep the person calm and encourage them to rest.

3. Choking:

Recognition:

- Difficulty breathing or speaking.
- Clutching the throat.
- Inability to cough or make a sound.

Response:

- Encourage coughing if the person can.
- If coughing is ineffective, perform the Heimlich maneuver (abdominal thrusts).
- Call emergency services if the obstruction persists.

4. Seizures:

Recognition:

- Uncontrolled shaking or convulsions.
- Loss of consciousness.

- Confusion after the seizure.

Response:

- Move objects away to prevent injury.
- Protect the person's head.
- Time the duration of the seizure.
- Call emergency services if the seizure lasts longer than 5 minutes or if another seizure follows immediately.

5. Allergic Reactions (Anaphylaxis):

Recognition:

- Swelling of the face, lips, or tongue.
- Difficulty breathing.
- Rapid or weak pulse.

Response:

- Administer an epinephrine auto-injector if available.
- Call emergency services.

6. Diabetic Emergencies:

Recognition:

- Confusion or irritability.
- Rapid breathing or shortness of breath.
- Changes in level of responsiveness.

Response:

- If conscious, provide sugar (candy, juice, or glucose gel).
- If unconscious, call emergency services.

7. Fainting (Syncope):

Recognition:

- Sudden loss of consciousness.
- Pallor and sweating.

Response:

- Lay the person down and elevate their legs.
- Ensure a supply of fresh air.

General Guidelines for Responding to Medical Emergencies:

- Call for Help: Dial emergency services immediately.

- Stay Calm: Keep yourself and others calm to facilitate effective response.

- Provide Comfort: Reassure the person and keep them as comfortable as possible.

- Do Not Leave Unattended: Stay with the person until professional help arrives or the situation resolves.

Remember that these guidelines are general in nature, and specific situations may require variations in response. It is highly recommended to seek professional training in first aid and CPR to enhance your ability to recognize and respond to medical emergencies effectively.

Fire safety and evacuation

Fire security and departure arranging are significant components to guarantee the well-being of people and communities within the occasion of a fire crisis. Here are key rules for fire security and departure.

Guarantee that your domestic is prepared with smoke alerts on each level and interior rooms. Test these cautions month to month and supplant batteries at slightest once a year. Distinguish essential and auxiliary elude courses from each room, and hone fire drills routinely, particularly in families with children.

Keep fire quenchers in key zones of the domestic, such as the kitchen and carport. It's important that everybody within the family knows how to utilize a fire quencher successfully. When cooking, never take off the stove unattended, and keep combustible things absent from cooking apparatuses. Frequently assess and keep up electrical apparatuses and wiring, and dodge over-burdening electrical outlets and control strips.

For warming gear, keep space radiators at slightest three feet absent from combustible materials, and guarantee that chimneys and warming gear are cleaned and reviewed frequently. When utilizing candles, put them in steady holders and keep them absent from combustible materials. Never take off candles unattended.

On the off chance that conceivable, smoke exterior and utilize profound, strong ashtrays. Guarantee cigarette butts are completely quenched. Store combustible fluids in endorsed holders absent from warm sources, and arrange of sleek clothes and other combustible materials securely.

In terms of departure arranging, guarantee everybody knows the nearby crisis number and have a list of crisis contacts promptly accessible. Set up assigned assembly focuses exterior your domestic and within the neighborhood. Make a communication arrange with family individuals and neighbors, assigning a central contact individual exterior the range.

Be commonplace with essential and elective clearing courses in your region for both vehicle and foot clearing. Plan an crisis pack with basics such as water, non-perishable nourishment, solutions, to begin with help supplies, and imperative reports. Keep the unit in an effectively open area. Arrange for the clearing of people with extraordinary needs, counting newborn children, elderly family individuals, or those with versatility challenges.

Conduct customary clearing drills along with your family, practicing diverse courses and assembly focuses. Remain educated around neighborhood fire dangers and clearing orders, tuning in to crisis alarms and taking after official informational. Incorporate pets in your clearing arrange, guaranteeing they have recognizable proof and considering their needs in your crisis unit.

Take an interest in community fire security programs and lock in with neighbors to cultivate a collective approach to departure arranging. By executing these fire security and clearing measures, people and communities can upgrade their readiness and strength within the confront of a fire crisis. Normal surveys and upgrades to the arrange guarantee its viability over time.

Emergency communication

Successful crisis communication is vital in guaranteeing the security and well-being of people and communities amid emergency circumstances. Clear communication channels must be set up in progress, including official crisis administrations, community pioneers, and significant specialists. The utilize of different devices, such as open address frameworks, sirens, and advanced stages, makes a difference spread basic data.

The issuance of crisis cautions and notices is vital for opportune communication with the open. Leveraging content messages, sirens, social media, and other stages guarantees that imperative data comes to individuals expeditiously. Considering the differences of communities, messages ought to be communicated in numerous dialects, and available groups like braille, sound, or expansive print ought to be given for people with inabilities.

Consistency in informing over distinctive channels is basic to maintain a strategic distance from disarray or clashing data that might lead to freeze or deception. Locks in with the community through associations, two-way communication, and inclusion of neighborhood pioneers cultivates successful communication amid crises.

Instruction plays a imperative part in planning the open to get and react to crisis communications. Conducting preparing sessions and drills familiarizes people with communication methods, upgrading their capacity to explore emergency circumstances. Innovation, counting crisis notice apps and social media, offers real-time communication openings, whereas conventional media outlets such as radio and tv can be utilized for broader reach.

Keeping up official government websites with up-to-date crisis data, setting up crisis hotlines, and observing social media for real-time overhauls are indispensably components of successful crisis communication. Post-emergency communication is similarly vital, giving upgrades on recuperation endeavors, accessible assets, and back administrations to the community.

Routinely investigating and overhauling crisis communication plans based on lessons learned from past occurrences, as well as looking for criticism from the community, guarantees persistent change. In outline, compelling crisis communication requires coordination, arranging, flexibility, and a commitment to straightforwardness to upgrade open security and reaction amid basic circumstances.

Dealing with natural disasters

Dealing with a natural disaster can be a difficult and overwhelming experience. Here are some important steps to deal with and deal with these situations.

1.   Stay informed: Stay informed of potential threats and evacuation orders by monitoring local news, weather information, and official sources. Follow affiliated organizations on social media for real-time updates.

2.   Create an emergency plan: Create an emergency plan for yourself and your family. Identify evacuation routes, create a communication plan, and designate a meeting point. Make sure everyone knows what to do in different scenarios and conduct regular training.

3.   Prepare an emergency kit: Stock up on essentials such as non-perishable food, water, first

aid kit, flashlight, batteries, blankets, and important documents. Keep your kit easily accessible and replenish it regularly.

4. Protect Your Home: Take preventive measures like securing heavy furniture, trimming trees, securing loose items, and reinforcing doors and windows. Consider installing storm shutters, reinforcing your roof, or investing in flood barriers if you live in a high-risk area.

5. Evacuation: If authorities issue an evacuation order, follow it promptly. Gather necessary items and essentials, including medications, important documents, cash, and clothing. Use designated evacuation routes and listen to official instructions.

6. Stay Safe During the Event: If you are unable to evacuate or seek shelter, find a secure area in your home away from windows and doors. Stay tuned to emergency broadcasts, remain calm, and use caution when using candles or generators.

7.   After the Disaster: Once it's safe to do so, assess your immediate surroundings for potential hazards. Check on your family and neighbors, and let others know you are safe. Avoid entering damaged buildings, fallen power lines, or floodwaters.

8.   Seek Assistance: Reach out to local authorities, disaster relief organizations, or emergency hotlines for assistance, information, and support in the aftermath of a disaster. They can provide guidance on recovery resources, shelter, and medical aid.

9.   Take Care of Emotional Well-being: It's normal to experience stress, anxiety, or trauma after a natural disaster. Take care of your emotional well-being by seeking support from family, friends, or professional counselors. Stay connected with others and engage in activities that promote self-care and resilience.

Remember, preparation is key to effectively dealing with natural disasters. Stay informed, have a plan in place, and take proactive steps to protect yourself, your loved ones, and your property.

Home emergency kit essentials

When putting together a home emergency kit, it's important to include essential items that can help you and your family during a crisis.

Here is a list of important items to consider:

1.   Water: Store at least 1 gallon of water per person per day for at least 3 days. It is recommended that all family members have enough water for her for 3 days.

2.   Non-perishable foods: Choose non-perishable foods that are easy to store and provide nutrition in an emergency. Examples include canned goods, muesli bars, nuts, dried fruit, and instant meals.

3.   First Aid Kit: The includes a fully stocked first aid kit with bandages,   tape, disinfectant,

painkillers, antihistamines, gloves, scissors, and all necessary prescription medications.

4.   Flashlights and Batteries: Have some flashlights with extra batteries.

5.   Choose an LED flashlight that is energy efficient and has a long lifespan

6.   Portable Radio: Receive important emergency alerts and updates during power outages with a built-in battery-powered or hand-crank radio.

7.   Additional Batteries: Keep additional batteries of various sizes on hand to power emergency equipment such as flashlights, radios, and other critical equipment.

8.   Blankets and Warm Clothing: Bring thermal blankets and sleeping bags to stay warm during power outages or when heating is not available. Also, please bring warm clothing appropriate for your local weather conditions.

9.   Personal hygiene products: This includes items such as toilet paper, wet wipes, hand sanitizer, toothbrushes, toothpaste, feminine hygiene products, and other personal care items specifically tailored to your needs

10.   Prescription Medications: Make sure you have an adequate supply of prescription medications for your entire family.

11.   Consider   taking   over-the-counter medications to relieve common ailments and pain.

12.   Copies of important documents: Keep copies of important documents, such as ID cards, insurance policies, medical records, and emergency contact information, in a waterproof, easily accessible container.

13.   Smoke and Carbon Monoxide Alarms: Install and maintain working smoke and carbon monoxide alarms in your home. Check the battery regularly and have a replacement battery available

14.   Fire Extinguisher: Keep a fire extinguisher in an easily accessible location and make sure all family members know how to use it. Understand the different types of fire extinguishers and their specific uses.

15.   Dust Mask or N95 Mask: When air quality is poor due to smoke, dust, or pollutants, it is important to wear a dust mask or N95 mask to protect your respiratory system.

16.   Protective Gloves: Includes heavy-duty work gloves to protect hands in emergency situations involving debris or potentially hazardous materials.

17.   Safety Glasses: Have safety glasses or goggles on hand to protect your eyes from dust, dirt, or potentially flying objects in an emergency.

18.   Reflective Vest or Reflective Tape: When evacuating or calling for help, wearing a reflective vest or using reflective tape on your clothing will

help you be more visible to rescuers and emergency personnel.

19.   Emergency Evacuation Plan: Prepare and practice an emergency evacuation plan for your home, including identifying multiple evacuation routes and a designated gathering area outside of your home.

20.   Emergency Contact List: Maintain a list of important emergency contact numbers such as local authorities, utility companies, medical professionals,   trusted family members and neighbors.

21.   Multi-Purpose   Tools: Contains multi-purpose tools or Swiss Army knives useful for a variety of emergency tasks.

22.   Extra Cash: Keep a small amount of cash on hand, as ATMs may not be available during power outages or other emergencies.

23.   Whistle: Add a whistle to call for help if you are trapped or need help.

24.   Mobile phone and portable charger: Make sure you have a fully charged mobile phone and a portable charger or power bank.

25.   Important Contact Information: Prepare a list of important contact numbers, such as emergency services, family, friends, and neighbors.

26.   Maps: Add local maps of your area and surrounding areas in case you need to choose a different route or evacuate.

Remember to periodically check and rotate items in your emergency kit to ensure food, water, and batteries are still usable. Additionally, consider including any items specific to your family's needs, such as baby supplies, pet essentials, or specialized medications.

It's also crucial to have a plan in place and educate your family members about the contents of the emergency kit, as well as the steps to take during an emergency. Stay informed about local emergency procedures and updates from official sources to ensure your family's safety.

Emergency situations can vary, so adapt your emergency kit contents accordingly.

Vehicle emergency preparedness

Being prepared for crises on the road is critical for both your own and others' safety. Here are some important things to have in your

1. automobile emergency kit: Spare tyre, jack, and lug wrench: Make sure you have a well inflated spare tyre and the equipment needed to fix a flat tyre.

2. Include jumper cables or a portable jump starter to restart your car in the event of a dead battery. Make sure you understand how to utilise them appropriately.

3. Reflective Warning Triangles or Flares: These may be put around your vehicle to alert other drivers and improve visibility, particularly at night or in low-visibility circumstance

4.   Tyre Pressure Gauge: Keep a tyre pressure gauge in your car to check tyre pressure on a regular basis and adjust as necessary. Properly inflated tyres are essential for safe driving.

5.   Include a basic toolkit consisting of screwdrivers, pliers, adjustable wrenches, and a pocket knife. These might assist you with small repairs and changes.

6.   Carry a multi-tool or emergency tool with capabilities such as a window breaker and seat belt cutter. These may be beneficial in the event of an accident or if you need to exit your car.

7.   Flashlight: Bring a flashlight with additional batteries or a rechargeable one that you can immediately reach in the event of a breakdown at night.

8.   Emergency Reflective Vest: If you need to escape your car at night or in high-traffic areas, wear a reflective vest to boost your visibility.

9.   Bottled water and non-perishable food, such as granola bars, should be kept on hand in case you get stuck for a lengthy period of time.

10.   Blanket or Sleeping Bag: If you are caught in cold weather, pack a blanket or sleeping bag to stay warm.

11.   First Aid Kit: Keep a basic first aid kit with bandages, antiseptic solution, pain medicines, and any personal drugs you may need.

12.   Roadside help Information: Keep your roadside help provider's contact information in your car, along with any membership details.

13.   Paper Maps: Keep paper maps of your neighbourhood and any locations you want to go through in case GPS or phone service is unavailable.

14.   Carry a portable phone charger or a vehicle charger to keep your phone charged and allow you to communicate in an emergency.

15. Keep a list of critical emergency contact numbers for family members, municipal authorities, and insurance companies.

Check and maintain your car emergency kit on a regular basis to verify that everything is in functioning shape and up to date. It's also a good idea to examine basic car maintenance and safety procedures so you're prepared to deal with any concerns that may emerge. Keep in mind that your geographic location and temperature might impact the things you need in your auto emergency kit. Customise your equipment to meet your specific demands and the circumstances in your location.

Water safety and drowning prevention

Water safety and drowning prevention are critical to saving lives, particularly in youngsters. Here are some important steps to increase water safety and avoid drowning

1. Supervision: Always keep children under careful supervision while they are near water, including pools, bathtubs, and natural bodies of water such as lakes or rivers. Adults should avoid distractions such as reading, phone use, or taking drink or drugs.

2. Learn to swim: Teaching children and adults how to swim is critical for water safety. Enrolling in swimming classes with experienced teachers may considerably lower the danger of drowning.

3.   Use life jackets: When sailing or engaging in water sports, be sure that everyone, particularly youngsters and novice swimmers, is wearing properly fitting life jackets. Life jackets should meet sufficient safety requirements.

4.   Securing pool areas: To prevent unsupervised access and limit the danger of drowning, install adequate barriers around pools, such as self-closing and self-latching gates.

5.   Learn CPR: Knowing cardiopulmonary resuscitation (CPR) may save lives in the case of a drowning. Taking a CPR certification course may help people prepare for emergencies.

6.   Be careful around natural bodies of water: Lakes, rivers, and seas may have unexpected circumstances, such as hidden currents and rapid dips. Always be careful and knowledgeable about the unique hazards and circumstances before swimming or participating in water sports.

7.   Educate children about water safety: Teach them about the hazards of being near water without supervision, the need of following safety standards, and how to call for assistance in an emergency.

These precautions, together with ongoing care and knowledge, may considerably minimise the danger of drowning and enhance water safety. The Centres for Disease Control and Prevention (CDC) and the American Red Cross are excellent sources for more information on water safety and drowning prevention.

Safety during power outages

1. During power outages, it is critical to prioritise safety to avoid accidents and reduce hazards. Here are some precautions to keep you safe during power outages

2. To reduce the danger of fire, replace candles with flashlights or battery-powered lanterns.

3. Unplug appliances and gadgets to avoid harm from power spikes when power is restored.

4. To avoid carbon monoxide poisoning, use a portable generator that is properly connected and positioned outside in a well-ventilated location away from windows and doors.

5. Refrigerators and freezers should be kept closed to keep food cold for extended periods of time.

6.   To prevent fire threats, use a well vented fireplace or wood-burning stove and keep the area well-maintained.

7.   Never use gas stoves or ovens for heating.

8.   Stay informed about the outage by listening to a battery-powered radio or staying connected via a mobile device.

9.   If required, utilise a power bank to recharge your phone for emergency communication.

10.   Avoid driving unless absolutely essential, since traffic lights and signals may not be working correctly.

Check on your neighbours, particularly the elderly or fragile ones, to guarantee their safety.

Remember to always be prepared for power outages by keeping emergency supplies such as flashlights, batteries, non-perishable food, and drinking water on hand.

Conclusion

To summarise, the significance of daily safety cannot be emphasised. Throughout this book, we've covered a variety of safety topics that are important to our everyday lives. The need for awareness, planning, and proactive actions emerges as a common issue across home, personal, internet, and occupational safety.

Everyday safety involves taking simple but major efforts to safeguard ourselves and others around us. It entails being aware of possible dangers and taking appropriate actions to avoid accidents and injuries.

We've discussed the need of having a secure home environment, protecting our belongings, and learning fire safety measures. We've emphasised the significance of driving safely, following traffic regulations, and avoiding distractions.

Furthermore, this book has highlighted the necessity of personal safety, such as being watchful in public places, trusting our instincts, and being wary of possible hazards. We've spoken about the necessity of good cybersecurity procedures for protecting ourselves in the digital realm, as well as preserving our physical and mental health.

Overall, daily safety is a shared duty. It needs each person to actively promote safety in their communities, companies, and homes. We can make our communities and ourselves safer by remaining educated, participating in continuous learning, and adopting a proactive mentality.

Let this book serve as a warning to not take safety for granted. It is an ongoing activity that should be included into our everyday routines and decision-making processes. By prioritising safety in our daily lives, we may reduce risks, avoid accidents, and enjoy happier, healthier lives.

Remember that safety is an attitude that should be nurtured and practiced on a daily basis. Let us embrace the ideals outlined in this book and make safety a high priority in all areas of our life. Together, we can build a safer and more secure future for everyone.

www.ingramcontent.com/pod-product-compliance
Lightning Source LLC
Chambersburg PA
CBHW051708250726

48653CB00007B/2926